The Complete

Codependency Guide for Beginners

How to Conquer Codependency, Set Boundaries, and Enjoy Healthy Relationships with Partners, Friends & Family

Ryan Deluca

Table of Contents

Introduction

I want to thank you and congratulate you for purchasing the book, *"Codependency Guide for Beginners: How to Conquer Codependency, Set Boundaries, and Enjoy Healthy Relationships with Partners, Friends & Family"*.

This book contains proven steps and strategies on how to reclaim your life and conquer codependency. It will help you eliminate codependency and its dangerous effects to your life and sanity. It also contains tips and strategies on how you can increase your self- esteem and set healthy personal boundaries that people must respect.

If your life is derailing because of codependent relationships, then this book is a must-read for you. This book will help you manage your relationships and turn codependent relationships into healthy, loving and symbiotic relationships.

If you feel like your life is in a downward spiral because of codependency, then it is time to take control of the situation and deal with it head on. With the help of this book, you will be able to understand codependency, its underlying causes and how to conquer it by addressing its root causes.

When you follow the tips and techniques contained in this book, you will be surprised with the positive changes in your life. You will be amazed with how your life will take a positive turn. Be happy and free from worry. Learn to fulfill your personal dreams and live your life to the fullest.

Thanks again for purchasing this book, I hope you enjoy it!

Please take some time to stop by and LIKE our Facebook page:

https://www.facebook.com/joypublishing

With gratitude,

Ryan Deluca

Chapter 1

ABCs of Codependency

We encounter the word "codependent" all the time – in newspapers, TV shows, self-help books, psychology textbooks or in our everyday conversations. It is often used to describe a person who is weak, dependent, easily manipulated and who has relationships with people who take advantage of them.

If you suspect that you are codependent, it is necessary to know and be familiar with its symptoms and causes. It is also necessary to learn strategies and techniques that you can use to put an end to codependency and reclaim your life.

Definition and History of the Term "Codependency"

Codependency was first coined in the 1980s to describe couples who are both dependent on alcohol and illegal drugs. The term actually came from the group Alcoholics Anonymous (AA) when its members discovered that the families of alcoholics and drug addicts usually had a common behavioral pattern that affected those who suffered from substance abuse. This idea is the foundation of the term "codependency" which initially described a person's preference to be in a relationship with partners who were dependent on substances or chemicals.

However, the meaning of codependency has since evolved due to the studies that have been done in the recent years. Codependency is now defined as a toxic relationship or a psychological condition where a person is being controlled and manipulated by another person who suffers from pathological conditions such as alcohol addiction, drug addiction or narcissism. Generally a codependent person is described as a person who is fixated on another person for sustenance, approval and so on.

Codependency is used to describe a set of behaviors, feelings and thoughts that go far beyond the normal boundaries of care-taking or self-sacrifice. Take a parent, for example. Generally, parents are expected to care for their children and give them emotional and financial support. However, there are parents who sacrifice too much for their kids. Their self-sacrifice is unhealthy and destructive. A codependent parent can be harmful to his/her child and his/her parenting style is less effective.

A codependent person routinely puts other people's needs and desires before their own. They are often the "mother hen" of a certain group and they take on responsibilities that are not even theirs. In doing this, they often forget about their own needs and desires since they often crave for acceptance and they always want to feel needed. They feel uncomfortable, restless and depressed when they do not feel needed. A codependent person does not stand up for himself and feels guilty whenever he does.

However, if you are a naturally caring and nurturing person, it does not automatically mean that you are codependent. Codependency only happens when caring, sacrificing, and providing for another person is excessive, unhealthy, and destructive.

Effects of Codependency

People who are in codependent relationships resort to self-destructive behavior to feel better about their selves. They often binge-eat until they are obese. They shop recklessly until they are drowned in debt. In most cases, they often develop an addiction to alcohol and drugs. Some codependent people often resort to promiscuity and reckless sexual behavior just to feel accepted and loved. Other codependent people work excessively to numb their feelings and silence their pain. Some even gamble excessively and uncontrollably until they eventually get into different sorts of financial problems.

Codependent people often refuse to acknowledge that something is wrong in their relationships. They avoid conflict and refuse to stand up for themselves. Because of this, they seek affirmation, validation, and pleasure elsewhere – work, expensive purchases, gambling and promiscuous affairs.

Codependent relationships or marriages may be harmful to the children as well. It is only natural that children learn behavior and responses from the adults around them, particularly their parents. When children are exposed to a codependent relationship, they might grow up with low self-esteem. They may also lack the integrity that is necessary in maintaining healthy adult relationships. These children may grow up unable to say no to a demanding boss or an abusive romantic partner.

Causes of Codependency

Most codependent people come from dysfunctional families. They learned these codependent behaviors from their parents or other members of their family. These kids are often exposed to a family member or relative who is addictive, compulsive or has a mental disorder. Long-term exposure to codependency is deemed to be the primary cause of the development of codependent behavior. Studies show that people who are exposed to codependent behavior develop a culture of distrust, controlling behavior, hypervigilance, denial and stress issues. Studies also show that people become codependent through living and being in a family with rules that prevents flexibility, spontaneity, and development. Here are some of the rules imposed by a codependent person's parent that could cause the development of codependent behavior:

1. Never trust other people, not even your own instincts.

2. You should never talk about problems.

3. You should keep your feelings to yourself.

4. Do not be selfish. You have to put other people's needs first.

5. It is not okay to be rowdy, joyful, and playful.

6. You have to pretend like there are no problems at all.

7. Always be strong, good, and perfect.

8. Do not ever rock the boat.

9. You should feel guilty each time you say "no". Therefore, never say no.

10. Do everything to make your parents proud.

11. Always guard and keep family secrets.

12. You should control things and people to feel safe.

13. Do not do anything to disgrace your parents.

14. Do not openly express unpleasant feelings.

These rules when rigidly imposed in a family could suppress the person's ability to stand for himself and for what he believes is right. A person who belongs to a family with these sets of rules will most likely do everything in their power to please their loved ones and to make sure that he does not disappoint them. This can be the root of a codependent behavior which he may develop later on.

The educational system and religious beliefs could also contribute to the development of codependent behavior. We are all taught in school and in church to be a "good person" and to "put other people's needs first". Most religious institutions even praise and encourage martyrdom.

The media also plays a vital part of the development of codependency. Self-sacrifice and being a martyr is somehow romanticized in movies and other forms of fiction.

Codependent behavior is very dangerous. It could destroy a person's ability to live life on his own terms and fulfill his dreams and desires. It is important for you to recognize what a codependent behavior is. Sadly, most codependent people think that these behaviors are normal and are even applauded for these behaviors. However, codependent behavior is certainly not normal and it should be dealt with as soon as possible.

Chapter 2

Are you a Codependent Person and Are You in a Codependent Relationship?

Here are the characteristics of a codependent person:

1. Codependent people have very low self-esteem and self-worth – Codependent people do not see their value. They always feel that they are not good enough and they also feel the need to compare themselves to others. But here's the tricky thing about people who have low self-esteem, on the outside, they appear confident, capable, beautiful and worthy. They have good posture, they may hold an important position in a company, and they may be very eloquent. But deep inside, people who have low self-esteem feel inadequate and unloved. Underneath, they feel shame and guilt. People who are perfectionists often have low self-esteem. They may appear confident and proud of their abilities and skills, but perfectionism is just their ploy to make them feel good about themselves.

2. Codependent people always aim to please others – It is normal to have a desire to please the people that you love and care about. However, codependent people take people-pleasing to the next level. Codependent people are unable to say "no" even if they want to because they do not want to disappoint anyone. They become anxious each time they say "no" to people they care about. Most co-dependents have a hard time saying "no" to almost anyone. They

always accommodate other people's wants and needs that they often forget their own.

3. Codependent people have poor boundaries – A boundary is basically an imaginary line between you and another person. It separates what is yours from the things that belong to other people. Boundaries apply to your body, property, money, thoughts, needs and feelings. The problem with codependent people is that they have difficulty setting up healthy boundaries between them and other people. They feel responsible for other people's dreams, feelings and problems. They take responsibility of things that they are not responsible for and they often give unsolicited advice. They tolerate behaviors that are otherwise unacceptable and they allow other people to continually hurt their feelings. Because codependent people have poor boundaries, they have a tendency to take everything personally.

Codependent people often neglect themselves and their own problems in order to take care of other people and help them with their problems, difficulties and concerns. It is natural to feel empathy and sympathy. And yes, it is great if you want to help other people out of the goodness of your heart. But the problem with codependent people is that they start putting other people's needs and wants ahead of their own. Codependent people often feel rejected if the people they love do not want any help. They often feel the responsibility to "fix" the people they love.

4. Codependent people take everything personally – Codependents have a tendency to take everything personally. They react to other people's feelings, emotions

and opinions. Because they do not have boundaries, they feel that the opinions and feelings of the people they love somehow have to do with them.

5. Codependent people try their best to control people and situations – All of us want to have a feeling that we are in control. At some point, all of us feel that it is best if we have control over certain situations because we do not want to live our lives in uncertainty. That is actually normal. But for codependent people, the need and desire to control limit their ability to share their feelings to others and take necessary risks. Codependent people feel safe whenever they are in control. This is the reason why they try their best and do whatever it takes to control any situation. Codependent people often become alcoholics and workaholics to make them feel relaxed and in control. They need to control other people's behavior to feel okay and to feel secure. Codependents actually use people-pleasing and caretaking to manipulate the people close to them and make them act in a certain manner.

6. Codependents have an inclination to be dependent – Codependents have this huge need for people to like and value them. Well, at some point, everyone wants to be liked. But, codependent people want other people to like them so bad that this desire often drives them to subdue their own identity and resort to people-pleasing. They are afraid of being abandoned or being rejected by the people they care about. Most codependents feel that they should constantly be in a relationship because they feel sad, alone and depressed if they are on their own for a long period of

time. This is the reason why most codependents have a hard time ending an abusive and unhealthy relationship.

7. Codependents often have different kinds of painful emotions – Codependency often leads to stress, anxiety, depression, hopelessness, anger, bitterness and other difficult emotions. They often experience shame and they are in ceaseless awe of being turned down or given up. They are also often afraid of being judged by the people they care about. Codependents feel these painful emotions almost all the time. This is the reason why codependents often become emotionally dead.

8. Codependents are often in denial – It is somewhat hard to convince a codependent to get assistance because most codependents do not want to confront the trouble. They do not want to admit that there is a problem and something has to be done about it. They often blame others and they do not want to accept that something is really wrong with them. Codependents also frequently deny their real feelings, needs, wants and desires. Because they deny their feelings often, eventually they will have a hard time identifying their own needs and emotions. So, they often focus on other people's wants, desires, needs and dreams. Codependents have trouble receiving love, support and even material things.

9. Codependents often have a problem with intimacy – Although some codependents may have problems with sexual intimacy; most of them have a problem with emotional intimacy. They find it hard to be open and emotionally vulnerable to the people they love. They usually feel intense shame and they do not expose

themselves emotionally because they are afraid of being rejected or judged.

10. Codependents are often dishonest – Codependents are often dishonest with themselves. But, it is important to take note that they are also often dishonest to others. They resort to lying because they are afraid of being judged and they are afraid of rejection.

11. Codependents are often obsessed with other people's feelings and relationships – Because codependents have poor boundaries, they are often obsessed with other people's feelings and affairs. They spend a lot of time thinking about other people or their own relationships. They examine every detail, behavior and response. They are often obsessed about the mistakes that they have made and the things they could have done. Codependents often have fantasies about how they want things to be. This is their way of staying in denial and escape reality.

12. Codependents have difficulty in communicating their feelings and opinions – Codependents often have a hard time communicating their feelings and preferences to the people they love. Codependents are afraid of being honest and truthful because they do not want to upset or disappoint the people they care about. They often pretend to like something that they really don't in order to please and manipulate other people.

Are You in a Codependent Relationship?

You may be wondering if you are in a codependent relationship. If you suspect that your relationship is indeed codependent then you need to do this – ask yourself what you really want in life. What are your dreams, goals and desires? If your answer depends on your partner and what he wants, then you must be in trouble.

Also, ask yourself what you think about certain situations or concepts like sex, money or having kids. If your answer is always tied to the opinion, preference and views of your partner, it could be an indication that you are in a codependent relationship. In a codependent relationship, one of the partners is unable to set boundaries or even say no. This is the reason why a codependent relationship is often not mutually respectful.

Here are some of the indicators that you are in a codependent relationship:

1. You are frequently afraid to say what you think or feel because of your fear of being abandoned.

2. Your opinions and views are often tied to the opinion and views of your partner.

3. You are constantly afraid to ask for what you want.

4. You feel guilty when you ask for what you want or when you say no.

5. You can't be open about how you feel.

6. Your partner always makes all the major decisions.

7. You feel the need to control and manipulate your partner but, at the same time, you also feel that you are being controlled or manipulated.

8. You feel trapped.

There are typically two types of people in a codependent relationship – the codependent or the giver and the partner who has a pathological condition or the taker. People who are immensely attracted to codependents are those who are addicted to alcohol, drugs or those who have serious personality disorders and narcissistic tendencies. The takers often have no boundaries. They see the codependent as an extension of themselves. They always require their codependent partner to be on-call to fulfill their wants, preference and needs. They do not care if the "giver" is in pain or ill. The need of the "takers" is endless, whether it's admiration, material commodity, flattery or emotional support.

Narcissists are often attracted to codependents and codependents are often attracted to narcissists. This is because narcissists are in constant need of someone who will do anything to fulfill their needs. Codependents, on the other hand, are in constant need of approval. They have an immense desire to fulfill someone else's needs.

A codependent relationship is very dangerous and can cause different sorts of problems even outside your relationship. It can affect your career, your personal development, and even your relationships with your friends and other family members. If you are a codependent who is constantly being taken advantage of or abused by your narcissistic partner, then it is high time to conquer codependency and take control of your life.

Chapter 3

Conquering Codependency

Codependency may lead to different long term problems such as depression, low self-esteem, health problems, career problems and relationship difficulties. Co-dependents often feel trapped, abused and they often feel that they are unable to trust anyone.

But there is hope. If you are a codependent, it is not too late. You can either end a codependent relationship or shape it to become more healthy and balanced. You can still reclaim your life and take control.

Here are the steps on how you could conquer and cure codependency:

- Acknowledge that there is a problem – Codependents are constantly in denial. They routinely deny that they have a problem. The first step in conquering codependency is to acknowledge it. You have to accept the fact that there is a problem. Be realistic. Realize that the relationships that you are in are not balanced. You have to recognize that the people you care about are taking advantage of you- your friends, family, spouse, kids, siblings or parents. Once you acknowledge and accept this, then you are on your way to recovery.

- Make a decision to do whatever it takes to conquer codependency – You have to make a tough decision to wage a war against codependency. After you have acknowledged that codependency is your problem, this is the time to decide to take steps that are necessary to end your codependency and make your life better. This is very difficult to do, but once you have made up your mind and you made the commitment to make positive changes in your life, there is no turning back. Everything will eventually become easier, lighter and you will be genuinely happy and feel more fulfilled.

- Get some help – It is necessary to talk to someone you trust about your codependency and the steps that you will take to end it. You can talk to an emotionally healthy family member or friend or you could see a mental health professional. You can also seek the help of spiritual leader that you respect and you can trust. The support of the people around you will push you into the direction of recovery.

- Focus on yourself – This is very important. If you want to conquer codependency, you have to focus on your own needs, wants and dreams. Take time to ask yourself – what do I really want? If you find yourself answering based on what your partner wants, ask yourself again and again until you get the real answer. If you are a codependent, you have spent so much time and effort focusing on other people's wants and needs that you have already forgotten your own desires and needs. Now is the time to be in touch with your own needs and your own desire. Do you want to go back to school or start your own business or maybe travel around the world? Acknowledge your needs, feelings, emotions and your dreams.

- Practice Self-Love – Self-love is not the same with narcissism. In fact, narcissistic people may appear confident on the outside, but deep inside, they despise themselves and feel inadequate. People who love themselves, on the other hand, accept themselves unconditionally. They do not take abuse and disrespect. They do not take advantage of other people and they do not allow others to take advantage of them. They are more direct in communicating their needs and their preference. While they clearly communicate their wants, desires, opinions and views, people who profoundly love themselves tend to respect other people's wants, needs and opinions. They do not judge others and they do not feel that they should change or fix other people. More importantly, people who constantly practice self-love have healthy boundaries. They do not allow people to meddle with their lives and they do not meddle with other people's lives. When you accept yourself completely, you do not have the urge or need to be accepted by others. Here's how you can practice self-love:

1. Say positive affirmations every morning – Positive affirmations can do wonders in your life. It can fill your life with love and happiness. You can find several affirmations online or you could make your own affirmations.

2. Take time to meditate – Meditation shuts off negative energy and allows you to focus on the positive.

3. Enjoy life – If you are a codependent, you have spent so much time taking care of other people that you have already forgotten to take care of yourself. Enroll in a yoga class, dance class or travel. Go to the beach often, if that's what makes you happy. Take time to hang out

with your old friends and take time to go to dinner parties.

4. Learn something new – Expand your skills and make yourself better. You can learn a new language or learn how to play guitar, crochet or you can go to pottery class. You can also visit the local museums and libraries. Go back to business school if that's what you want or get a master's degree. Follow the desires of your heart.

5. Live in gratitude – To be happy, you have to appreciate whatever it is that you have. Take time to appreciate and be grateful for your job, family and life in general. Savor that plate of baked macaroni. Stop and appreciate the view. Be grateful and you will no longer feel the need to manipulate or to let others take advantage of you just to be happy.

6. Always do the things and actions that honor you and respect you – Do not ever allow abusers and toxic people in your life. Do not engage with people who bring you down. Do not participate in activities that are harmful to you.

7. Believe in your self-worth – Understand that your worth is not dependent on someone's approval. You have to know and understand that you are worthy of love and respect. Once you realize your own self-worth, you will be surprised with how your life will change in a positive way.

- Let go of the need to change and fix other people – To conquer codependency, you have to let go of your need to control other people's lives. You must let go of your need or desire to change other people. This is one of the powerful ways to heal and cure codependency. Allow people to be themselves and resist any urge to try to change them and make them better. This means that you have to stop the care taking, rescuing, controlling, apologizing and pretending. You have to also avoid making rules for other people.

- Create and define your personal boundaries- This is ultimately necessary if you want to conquer and cure your codependency. Personal boundaries are basically decisions that you make about the behaviors that you will and won't tolerate.

If you have weak boundaries, you will tolerate just about anything. You allow people to hurt you and disrespect you. You also inappropriately assume responsibility for other people's mistakes, problems and experiences. If you have strong boundaries, you know where your responsibility ends and where others responsibilities begin. You draw a line between your concerns and the concerns of others. You stand up for yourself and you communicate your displeasure when someone is being hurtful or disrespectful to you.

Remember that setting boundaries is not enough. You have to enforce them. You have to communicate your feelings openly and honestly and call out people who violate them.

Here are some easy steps on how you could create boundaries:

1. Decide what you will and will not tolerate. Take time to reflect and determine what behaviors are tolerable and what behaviors are absolutely unacceptable. Prepare a list of acceptable and unacceptable behaviors.

2. Watch and determine certain violations of your boundaries. Other people may not be aware that they are crossing your boundaries so it is important to communicate with others what your boundaries are. For instance, you do not want to take work related telephone calls during your day off. You must clearly communicate with your coworkers that you would appreciate it if they will not contact you on weekends about work-related matters.

3. Enforce your personal boundaries by calling out people who violate these boundaries. Respectfully but clearly communicate that you will not tolerate these kinds of behavior. Directly express your displeasure and then present a possible solution or alternative.

- Be true to yourself – Most co-dependents have completely forgotten about their needs and desires. You have to maintain your personal integrity and be completely honest about who you are, what your dreams are, and how you feel. To heal a relationship, you have to be completely honest and become more genuine. You also have to stop caring about what other people think of you. You just have to live in the moment. Realize that it is okay not to be perfect.

- Leave when you have to – Finally, when you think that you cannot change the course and the nature of your codependent relationship, it is time to leave and end the relationship. If you decide to end it, you have to end it in a healthy way. Experts say that a codependent relationship automatically ends whenever you stop responding to your partner in a codependent way. The relationship automatically ends when you set healthy boundaries and enforce it. Remember to avoid drama. Ending a codependent relationship should not be emotionally charged. Just stay calm and just communicate that if your partner could not respect your boundaries, wants and needs, then it is best to end the relationship.

Once you follow these steps, you will be surprised with the positive changes in your life. You will be happier. Your career will thrive. Your relationships will be healthier and you will be able to get rid of the diseases associated with codependency like depression, anxiety, and emotional pain. You will be able to travel more, eat in restaurants that you really like and pick out the clothes that you prefer. You will feel empowered and confident. In no time, your confidence will reach its all-time high and you can now put your painful, codependent past behind you.

Chapter 4

Rebuilding Your Life

Rebuilding your life is going to be one of the hardest things you ever have to do, but it will also be one of the most fulfilling. Working your way to a goal of self-fulfillment, a sense of inner peace and all-around good health will be an amazing accomplishment that you will surely be proud to have reached. This is not going to be any kind of quick fix but it will be a work in progress throughout your lifetime. Find positive stepping stones to use in reaching a healthier way of life. Each progressive stone will get you one step closer to reaching all of your goals.

Overcoming Guilt and Resentment

Guilt is a possible persistent source of pain. Codependent people keep on reminding themselves to condemn who they are, live with guilt and end up destroying themselves. This guilt brings anger and resentment, not only to themselves but also to people around them.

Sometimes, guilt is good. Guilt can make people empathize, take the right course of action and to make themselves better individuals. After guilt, forgiveness of one's self should always follow as it is an essential key to life and relationships. For many, however, self-acceptance still remains hard to get hold of due to unhealthy guilt, and this guilt can stay with a person for years, decades, or even for a lifetime.

Why should negative feelings such as guilt, resentment and anger be avoided? One, they drain you of all your energy. Two, they bring illness and depression. Three, they prevent you from having happiness and having successful and fulfilled relationships. They hinder you from moving on and stop you from moving forward.

Codependents usually have guilt within them. It's common for them to accept the blame and feel responsible for another's wrongdoings because of their lack of self-esteem. Guilt, however, should be differentiated with shame. Shame is when you feel inadequate and inferior and makes you tend to underestimate yourself and your relationships.

How do you overcome these feelings of shame, guilt and resentment? Ask these questions to yourself, and follow these steps.

- Take responsibility if you've been rationalizing your actions. Tell yourself, "Yes, I did it." Look back and remember what happened. Think about how you felt, and think about other people involved in the process. Consider what were your needs during those times, and if they were met. If those needs weren't met, then why weren't they? What were your motives in doing so? Was there any catalyst for such behavior? Is this catalyst connected to a person or an event in your past? You can write them all down with a dialogue that includes your feelings.

- While growing up, how were your feelings and mistakes handled? Were you judged for them? Punished? Forgiven? Were people hard on you because of those mistakes? Were you somehow made to feel ashamed?

- How do you judge yourself? Are they really based on your personal faith and principles, or are they based on someone else's approval? Do you still need someone else's support before you go for something that you like? Don't aim to live up on another person's expectations – there are instances on which you'll never get their approval, and in doing so, you might end up sacrificing your own happiness and wants.

- Are your current actions matched with your true values? If not, think of your thoughts, emotions and beliefs that made you do your actions. What may have led you to abandon your values? In violating your values, you end up hurting yourself, which is more painful than hurting someone else.

- How did these conflicts affect you and other people? Take note of those people that you've hurt, and remember that you've hurt yourself as well. Reflect on how you can make amends and ask forgiveness from these people. How can you make things better? Can you still do something to ease the pain?

- If someone did you wrong, you possibly forgive them easily. Why then would you treat yourself differently? Do you think it benefits you to punish yourself continually?

- There's nothing wrong with making mistakes as long as you learn from them. Remorse is acceptable – even healthy – and it leads to creating corrective action. You'll learn how to act differently. Write yourself a letter filled with appreciation, understanding and forgiveness. Repeat these words to yourself: *I forgive myself. I'm innocent. I love myself.*

- Surround yourself with people who won't judge you for your past. Share to them what you did. Avoid secrecy to avoid further prolonging guilt and shame.

What is a healthy and humble attitude? You believe you're at fault but you still forgive yourself. Others were wrong, yet you forgive them. You regret the things that happened in the past yet you understand it was just a part of being human, and you ended up learning from your mistakes and you gain experience.

Raising Your Self-Esteem

Self-esteem is an assessment of someone's worth, or how an individual judges himself. It's also defined as a person's competency in coping with life's basic challenges, and deserving of happiness. Low self-esteem is one of codependency's main symptoms, and it has to be addressed as soon as possible.

Codependents are often sensitive and are afraid of abandonment or rejection. The "esteem" they have is based on how others see them and perceive their character. They live by solving problems of other people and this boosts their morale in a distorted way. If something goes awry, they take the blame and bear the guilt. They fill up their schedule to focus on one person – they have this feeling of being needed, and this feeling overcomes everything else.

Codependents usually come from dysfunctional, troubled, or repressed families. They deny it, though, hence the failure of solving their personal issues brought by them being codependents.

They take the blame for almost everything yet also blame others for everything. They reject compliments but are saddened when they don't get complimented. They are scared of being rejected yet reject themselves. They don't think they will be loved or liked, so they tend to show others they are lovable enough to be accepted by other people.

How should you reclaim your self-esteem?

- Challenge any self-defeating thoughts or beliefs about self-worth. You don't have to confirm anything to anyone about yourself.

- See yourself in a loving relationship that fulfills your desires and meets your needs. If your present relationship is damaging, look at ways on how you self-sabotage and observe your own behaviors.

- Tell yourself every day that it's healthy to receive help from others, and it's an indication of strength rather than weakness. Friendships, counseling, and other online resources can be ultimately helpful to guide you in looking for a happy relationship.

- Become aware of any negative judgments you have about yourself. Don't be harsh; you have to be kind and compassionate on yourself.

- Don't be afraid of rejection; go ahead and get involved in intimate and loving relationships. Concede and let go of your shield, and allow others in your life.

Have you considered that you're just hooked on the pain brought by love? If yes, then remind yourself that you risk your chances of having happy and healthy relationships where your needs can be fulfilled. Are you afraid of being alone? Are you scared of taking a risk? If you are, then you are preventing yourself from seeking the happiness and love you deserve.

Focus on your healing and your personal growth and begin to transform your life and attract others who are in the same emotional level as you.

Separating Responsibilities

Another vital task that codependents have to understand is how to separate responsibilities for themselves and for others. They react on other people's concerns. As these problems become more intense, codependents' reactions are more intense as well. They tend to be more involved in the process, hence keeping them in a chaotic state, as well as the people around them. Their energies are focused on other people and their problems which make them less attentive to their own lives.

In rescuing others, codependents aim to take care of people who can perfectly live their own lives. They dwell on problems they don't have control over, and can be upset when things go wrong. What they don't know is that rescuing these people from their responsibilities doesn't help them grow but instead makes them evade the outcome of their actions more. Love makes codependents undertake in manipulative behavior. Their intentions are to help, and they end up being people who force things to happen using too much effort and energy.

Codependents fail to realize that other people don't need controlling, and these people would usually have no interest in

30

obtaining the outcome the codependent is aiming for. Codependents must understand as well that people will simply do what they wish to do regardless if they're wrong or right, or if they're hurting themselves.

Codependents who do other people's tasks do not help other people become better by rescuing them -- they instead teach them to be more dependent, and will lead to them to taking advantage of the codependent. In return, the codependent becomes resentful, overburdened, and ultimately vengeful and upset simply because they do things they don't wish to do.

Chapter 7

How to Recover from Codependency?

Recovery from codependency will need a lot of effort and determination from you. It might require you to make a 180-degree turnaround of the patterns that you have been used to. However, your healing will bring about strong characteristics that you can benefit from:

- You become authentic

- You become independent

- You open yourself to intimacy

- Your values, feelings, thoughts, beliefs and actions are aligned

In anything, change is difficult but it is good. There is no shortcut to being free from something that you have been accustomed to. Similar to recovery from any addiction, you have to overcome it.

Since change and recovery take time, the following techniques can help you:

- Your main goal is to bring the attention back to yourself. This doesn't mean becoming self-centered that you end up alienating your friends. Practice sobriety. You need the help of other people and they need your help too but you have to make sure that you make guided discernment. You can't say "yes" all the time as you cannot save the world. You learn to detach and you stop being too controlling.

This way, you begin to become independent and more self-oriented.

- Since codependency is a form of addiction, you need to stop denying and start becoming aware of the real problems. Codependents who are in abusive relationships endure the pain for fear of being alone; little do they know that they are slowly leading their lives into total destruction.

The first step to your recovery from codependency is to recognize that you are in a codependent relationship. Be aware of the signs and indications that you are in such a relationship. Regain your self-esteem by being true to yourself and admitting that there is a problem.

- Recovery involves acceptance. There is no shortcut to your recovery because it takes time and you have to be patient. Recovery and healing is a life-long journey that you have to take. However, before you can begin changing your life, you have to learn to accept your situation and accept that you need to make some life-changing decisions.

It takes a great level of maturity to learn to accept. When you are able to accept, you will be opening some new doors towards change, fresh ideas and renewed energy. These are doors you have long ignored because you have been living in a co-dependent relationship.

Aside from accepting the situation, you also need to accept yourself. Accept that you are not perfect and you have flaws. When you can accept yourself like that, you don't have to do whatever it takes to make people like you. When you emanate self-esteem and renewed confidence in

34

yourself, the right people will be drawn to you. They will be your true friends.

Acceptance teaches you to be more real and assertive. You begin to find out what you really want. You stop being too manipulating and you enjoy your relationships more because of the mutual respect and honest intimacy.

- Act on it. As most people say, insight without action can only get you so far. If you want to grow as a person and improve your life, you have to turn over a new leaf. You can't grow without taking risks. Get out of your comfort zone. Find your voice and use it well. Speak up and say what you want to say. Do not worry about what you will say; if it comes from the heart, it is sincere and true.

- If you have been in an abusive relationship for so long and you have in effect lost your freedom, try something new or go somewhere on your own.

- Do not rely on anybody to make you happy and fulfilled. Find your own happiness and fulfillment. Do the things that you've always wanted to do but you were just too afraid to do.

- Seek support. When you find yourself in a codependent relationship, you'll feel lost and confused at times. It's important to build a support network that you can fall upon in times of need. The wider your net, the better. Incorporate coworkers, friends, family, community resources, internet forums, etc. People trapped in relationships with addictions can find much comfort from programs such as Al-Anon. Al-Anon is an organization which offers support to friends and family of problem drinkers. However, there are many other programs that can be found in the community on a variety of different addictions.

- Accept the inevitable: you can't change the other person, you can only change yourself. This truth is at the core of all Al-Anon and other 12-step programs and is not just limited to these addiction recovery programs. This is true for all relationships regardless of how healthy or unhealthy. The Serenity Prayer, a prayer used in Alcoholics Anonymous, has become widely known throughout the North American culture. This prayer is commonly quoted in a variety of different circumstances in order to bring comfort and strength. Perhaps, you too will find comfort and strength from this famous prayer:

> *"God, grant me the serenity to accept the things I cannot change, the courage to change the things I can, and wisdom to know the difference"* (Reinhold Niebuhr).

When you regain confidence in yourself, you become empowered and more assertive. You begin to say what you really feel without offending other people. While you work on your relationships with other people, you shouldn't lose yourself in the process.

Avoiding a Relapse

When you begin your healing from codependency, you begin to feel your pain. Do not lose that pain, lest you fall back into being codependent. Listen to your pain and what it is telling you. Listen to your anger and know what it wants to convey to you.

You don't get out of a relationship that hurts you just so you will not be reminded of the pain you had to go through. Even if you get rid of the person, if you don't begin to heal yourself from within, you will always be vulnerable. Work on yourself and everything else will follow.

The Good Side of Codependency

You don't just get out of a codependent relationship by separating from your partner. It doesn't work that way. Instead of getting rid of the person, why not reconnect with yourself first?

Going back, your goal in overcoming a codependent relationship is to find yourself again. It got lost when you focused on pleasing other people so much that you forgot all about it. You can go through the process of healing without isolating yourself from the very people that you love. You just reconnect and reorganize your priorities.

Complete healing means you are able to live beyond the imperfection of your own personality and of humanity as a whole. You begin to see that living in a chaotic and dangerous world makes you vulnerable and you'll find strength in being true to yourself.

This knowledge and acceptance of who you are as a person will make you stronger and let you create more lasting relationships. The trick with relationships is to discover your joy and happiness regardless of the other person's thoughts, feelings and actions. The key is to understand your self-worth and set boundaries. This is true freedom from codependency.

Conclusion

Thank you again for purchasing this book! I hope this book was able to help you to help you understand codependency, its causes, its roots, and its symptoms. I also hope that this book was able to help you conquer codependency and live a better and healthier life.

The next step is to follow the tips, techniques, and strategies presented in this book. Reading this book is a huge step, but it is absolutely necessary to take action. You do not have to live a life of fear and unhappiness. You do not have to neglect your own needs and focus your energy on other people. This book has given you useful and easy to follow steps that will help you reclaim your life. It is time to do the dirty work and do the necessary steps to conquer your codependency.

Finally, please remember to LIKE our Facebook page in order to find other resources and upcoming promotions:

https://www.facebook.com/joypublishing

With sincere thanks,

Ryan Deluca

One Last Thing...

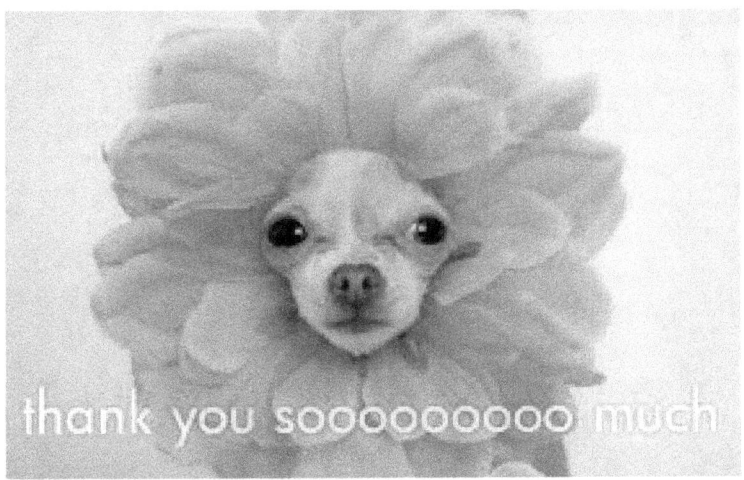

Source: Wikipedia

If you believe that this book is worth sharing, would you please take the time to let others on *Amazon* know how it affected your life? If it turns out to make a difference in the lives of others, they will be forever grateful to you, as will I.

www.ingramcontent.com/pod-product-compliance
Lightning Source LLC
Chambersburg PA
CBHW070507290526
45790CB00003B/1137